Get Fit Now

A Beginner's Guide to Exercising and Working Out

By

Charles Brooker

TABLE OF CONTENTS

1. Introduction to Exercise & Workouts

Welcome to the wonderful world of exercise and workouts! Exercise and workouts offer a variety of benefits that can improve your overall health and well-being. Regular physical activity helps you maintain a healthy weight, increases energy levels, reduces stress, strengthens bones and muscles, improves mental clarity and concentration, lowers blood pressure, and decreases the risk of heart disease, stroke, and other chronic diseases. Exercising doesn't have to be tedious; there are many fun ways to get moving such as running or walking outdoors in nature with friends or family members, joining an organized sports team, or taking up a new hobby like yoga or Pilates. Before starting any type of exercise program it is important to consult with your doctor first if you are pregnant or have any medical conditions. In this course, we will discuss different types of exercise and their benefits, how to get started with an exercise program, and the importance of warming up and cooling down. We will also explore various workout routines that can be tailored to fit your individual needs and goals.

Finally, we will discuss the importance of proper nutrition for optimal performance during workouts as well as tips on how to stay motivated to achieve success! Exercise and workouts can be a great way to improve your physical, mental, and emotional health. Whether you are looking for a fun way to stay active or want to take part in competitive sports, there is something out there for everyone! With the right knowledge and motivation, exercise can become an enjoyable activity that will help you reach your fitness goals. So let's get started on this journey together!

I.   Benefit of Exercise

1. Improved Cardiovascular Health: Exercise strengthens the heart muscle and improves the body's ability to deliver oxygen and nutrients to all cells, which can reduce your risk for a variety of illnesses, including heart disease and stroke. Regular exercise also helps to maintain healthy blood pressure levels.

2. Weight Management: Exercise is key when it comes to managing weight because it burns calories while building muscle mass. As you increase your muscle mass, you will burn more calories even at rest since muscles require energy to function properly.

3. Stronger Muscles & Bones: Exercise can help build strong bones as well as strengthen muscles by increasing their size, strength, and endurance over time. This can help reduce your risk of injury from everyday activities and improve your posture.

4. Improved Mental Health: Exercise can help to reduce stress, anxiety, and depression by releasing endorphins which trigger a positive feeling in the body. It can also help to boost self-esteem and confidence levels, as well as provide a sense of accomplishment from achieving goals or completing tasks that may have seemed daunting before beginning an exercise program.

5. Increased Energy Levels: Regular exercise helps to increase energy levels throughout the day by providing more oxygenated blood to all parts of the body including the brain

which helps you stay alert and focused for longer periods. This can be especially beneficial for those who suffer from chronic fatigue or low energy levels due to medical conditions such as fibromyalgia or diabetes.

6. Improved Sleep Quality: Exercise can help to regulate your body's natural sleep-wake cycle and improve the quality of your sleep by providing a better night's rest. This can be especially helpful for those who suffer from insomnia or other sleep disorders that make it difficult to fall asleep or stay asleep throughout the night.

7. Reduced Risk of Disease: Exercise can help to reduce your risk for a variety of diseases such as obesity, type 2 diabetes, osteoporosis, and certain types of cancer by increasing muscle mass and improving overall health. Additionally, it can help improve your immune system which will make you less susceptible to catching colds or other illnesses.

8. Improved Cognitive Function: Regular exercise can help to improve cognitive function, including memory and

concentration, by increasing the flow of oxygenated blood to your brain. This can be especially beneficial for those who are looking to sharpen their focus or boost their productivity at work.

9. Improved Flexibility: Exercise can help to increase your range of motion and improve flexibility, which will make it easier for you to perform everyday activities with ease. This is especially important as we age since our bodies tend to become less flexible due to reduced muscle mass and decreased joint mobility.

10. Better Mood: Exercise has been proven to be an effective way to reduce stress levels, improve mood and boost overall happiness by releasing endorphins that trigger a positive feeling in the body. It can also provide a sense of accomplishment when goals are achieved or tasks completed that may have seemed daunting before starting an exercise program.

II.   Types of Exercise

Exercise can be classified into four types:
1. Aerobic Exercise: These exercises involve large muscle groups and are performed for a sustained period, usually at least 20 minutes. Examples include running, swimming, biking, walking, and rowing. Aerobic exercise helps to strengthen your cardiovascular system by increasing your heart rate and breathing rate. It also increases the amount of oxygen in the blood which helps to improve overall health and fitness levels.
2. Strength Training: This type of exercise focuses on building muscle mass through resistance training such as weight lifting or bodyweight exercises like push-ups or pull-ups. Strength training can help increase bone density and reduce the risk of injury while also improving overall strength and power output during other physical activities.
3. Flexibility Exercises: These exercises are designed to increase the range of motion in your joints and muscles, helping you to

become more flexible and limber. Examples include stretching, yoga, and Pilates. Increased flexibility can improve performance in other physical activities as well as reduce the risk of injury due to tight or inflexible muscles or joints.

4. Balance Exercises: This type of exercise is important for maintaining a healthy body by improving balance, coordination, and stability while also reducing the risk of falls or injuries caused by poor posture or instability when performing other physical activities. Examples include tai chi, dancing, and various balance drills like single-leg squats or standing on one foot with eyes closed. In addition to these four main categories, other types of exercises can be beneficial for overall health and fitness such as core training, plyometrics, and interval training

III. Setting Goals For Yourself

Setting goals for yourself when it comes to exercise and working out can be an incredibly powerful tool. Goals are important because they provide focus, motivation, and a sense of accomplishment after achieving them. When setting goals related to physical activity, it is important to make sure that the goals are realistic and achievable for you to stay motivated and on track. Here are some tips for setting effective exercise goals:

1. Start by making your goal SMART – Specific, Measurable, Achievable, Relevant, and Time-Bound: Your goal should be specific enough so that you know exactly what needs to be done to achieve it. It should also have measurable outcomes so that you can track your progress toward reaching the goal. Make sure that your goal is achievable and realistic, so you don't get discouraged when trying to reach it. Additionally, make sure that the goal is relevant to what you are trying to achieve with your physical activity (e.g., lose weight or increase strength). Finally, give yourself a timeline by which

you want to accomplish the goal; this will help keep you on track and motivated towards achieving it.

2. Break down your main goal into smaller goals: It can be helpful to break down your main goal into smaller goals for them to seem more attainable and less overwhelming. This also helps create a sense of accomplishment as each small step brings you closer to reaching your final destination!

3. Set short-term and long-term goals: It is important to set both short-term and long-term goals, as this will help you stay motivated in the present while also keeping your eye on the prize. Short-term goals help stay focused on a day-to-day basis, while long-term ones will keep you motivated over a longer period.

4. Make sure that your goal is realistic and achievable: Setting an unrealistic goal can be discouraging when trying to reach it; instead, make sure that the goal is something that you know you can accomplish with some hard work and dedication.

5. Write down your goals: Writing down your goals makes them seem more tangible, which helps motivate you to reach them. Additionally, writing down your goals is an excellent way to track progress and stay on track toward reaching the goal.

Overall, setting goals related to physical activity can be a great way to stay motivated and focused on what you are trying to accomplish with exercise and working out. Make sure that your goals are SMART (Specific, Measurable, Achievable, Relevant, Time-Bound), break them down into smaller ones if needed for them to seem more manageable, and set both short-term and long-term goals so that you have something to work towards over time, make sure they are realistic and achievable so that you don't get discouraged when trying to reach them, and write them down so that you can track your progress and stay on track towards reaching the goal. With some hard work, dedication, and commitment to your goals, you will be able to successfully reach them in no time!

2. Getting Started With a Fitness Plan

Getting started with a fitness plan can be intimidating, especially if you are new to exercise or have been inactive for some time. However, it is important to remember that everyone starts somewhere and the most successful journey begins with small steps! Here are a few pointers to kick you off:

1. Set realistic goals - Setting achievable goals will help keep you motivated and make sure that your progress is steady and sustainable. Start by setting short-term goals such as attending an exercise class twice a week or running three miles twice per week. Once these become easier, increase the difficulty of the goal slightly so that you continue to challenge yourself while still making progress toward your end goal.

2. Find activities that you enjoy - Exercise should be something that you look forward to and enjoy, not dread. If jogging isn't for you, consider swimming or cycling. There are so

many activities out there – find one that works for you!

3. Find a buddy - Exercise is always more enjoyable when you have someone to do it with - it can help keep you accountable and motivated on days when it feels too hard to go alone.

4. Track your progress - Keeping track of how far or fast you have gone can be a great way to monitor your progress and stay motivated. Use an app if running or biking, or write down the weights used in each exercise during strength training sessions so that next time you know what weight to aim for.

5. Make it a habit - Exercise should be something that you make time for each week, just like brushing your teeth or doing the laundry. Make a note of it on your calendar and stick to it!

6. Take rest days - Rest is an important part of any fitness plan, as this is when your body recovers and gets stronger. Make sure that you take at least one day off per week so that your muscles can recover properly before the next session.

7. Reward yourself - Celebrate small successes along the way with non-food rewards such as a new piece of exercise equipment or clothing, or a massage to help with muscle recovery and soreness after tough workouts!

By following these tips and making exercise a part of your weekly routine, you will soon start to see results in terms of both physical and mental well-being.

I.   Choosing The Right Equipment

Choosing the right equipment for exercise and working out is an important step in achieving your fitness goals. The type of equipment you choose will depend on a variety of factors, such as what type of workout you are doing, how much space you have available, budget considerations, and personal preferences. When selecting exercise equipment, it's important to consider its safety features, adjustability options, and overall quality. You want something that can safely accommodate your body size and weight while also providing enough resistance or challenge to help progress your physical fitness level. In addition to these basic criteria, there are many other things to consider when choosing the right piece of equipment for your workouts:

1. Type Of Exercise: Determine which types of exercises you plan to do most often and select equipment that can accommodate them. For example, if you are mostly doing cardiovascular exercises like running or cycling, then a treadmill or stationary bike would be an ideal choice. On the other hand, if your focus is on strength training exercises such as weight lifting or bodyweight workouts, then free weights and adjustable benches are good options.

2. Space: If space is an issue for you, consider compact machines that don't take up too much room when in use. Many home gyms now offer a variety of pieces of equipment that can be folded away when not in use – perfect for smaller spaces! Also, think about how easily the machine can be moved around; some require more effort than others.

3. Budget: Exercise equipment can be expensive, so it's important to think about what you can realistically afford. Look for

good quality machines that are within your budget and come with a warranty in case of any issues. You may also want to consider second-hand or refurbished models if you're on a tighter budget – just make sure they still meet all safety requirements before making the purchase.

4. Features: When choosing exercise equipment, look for features that will help enhance your workout experience. For example, many treadmills now have built-in programs such as interval training and virtual running routes that can add variety and challenge to your workouts. Other features like adjustable inclines/declines, heart rate monitors, and iPod docks can also be beneficial.

5. Maintenance: It's important to consider the maintenance requirements of any exercise equipment you purchase. Look for machines that have easy-to-follow instructions and come with all the necessary tools for assembly, as well as regular cleaning and lubrication. Also, check if there are any additional parts or accessories you may need

to keep your machine functioning properly over time.

Overall, there are many factors to consider when selecting the right equipment for your exercise routine. Taking the time to research different options and compare features will help ensure you find something suitable for your specific needs and budget requirements. With the right piece of equipment in hand, you'll be well on your way toward achieving your fitness goals!

II. How Much You Should Exercise

Exercise is an important part of a healthy lifestyle, and how much exercise you should get depends on your age, health condition, and fitness goals. Generally speaking, adults should aim for at least 150 minutes of moderate-intensity aerobic activity or 75 minutes of vigorous-intensity aerobic activity each week. This can be broken down into shorter bouts throughout the day if that works better for your schedule. You should also add two days of strength training as well as flexibility and balance exercises to help keep your muscles strong and flexible.

For children ages 6 to 17, the American Heart Association recommends at least 60 minutes of moderate to vigorous physical activity per day—the more active they are during the day, the better their general health will be.

If you have a specific health condition or are recovering from an injury, you should consult with your doctor before starting any exercise program. They can help determine the best type of exercise for your needs and provide guidance on how much to do.

It's also important to remember that everyone is different and there is no "one size fits all" approach when it comes to exercise. It is recommended that people start slowly and build up their activity level over time as they become more fit. That way, they can find what works best for them in terms of intensity, duration, frequency, and type of activity without putting too much strain on their body at once.

Finally, it's important to listen to your body and not overdo it. If you're feeling sore or exhausted, take a break and focus on stretching or doing light activities like walking until you feel better. The key is finding the right balance of exercise that works for you so that you can stay active and healthy in the long run.

III. Creating Your Personalized Routine

Creating your personalized routine when beginning an exercise program can be a great way to set yourself up for success. Your routine should be tailored to your goals and needs, as well as the equipment you have available. Here are some tips for creating a workout routine that will work best for you:

1. Start slow – When starting, it's important not to push yourself too hard or too quickly. Begin with low-intensity activities like walking or biking and gradually increase intensity over time so your body can adapt and avoid injury. You may also want to consider consulting with a professional trainer who can help design a safe program specific to your fitness level and goals.

2. Choose exercises that fit your lifestyle– Consider what types of exercise you enjoy and can realistically fit into your daily schedule. If you don't like running, find other

activities that will get your heart rate up such as swimming or biking.

3. Vary the intensity– To achieve optimal results, it's important to mix up different intensities throughout your routine. This means alternating between high-intensity exercises like sprinting and low-intensity ones such as walking or jogging. Doing so will help keep your body challenged while avoiding overtraining and burnout.

4. Incorporate strength training – In addition to cardio exercises, add some strength training like weightlifting or resistance bands two to three times a week for optimal results. Not only does this help build muscle, but it also helps to improve your overall health and fitness level.

5. Make it fun – Exercise doesn't have to be a chore. Find activities that you enjoy such as dancing or team sports so that you look forward to your workouts instead of dreading them.

6. Track your progress– Use an app or journal to track the exercises you do each day, how long they took, and any other notes about how the

workout went (e.g., how challenging it was). This will help you stay motivated and make sure that you are making progress toward reaching your goals.

Creating a personalized workout routine can help you reach your fitness goals and stay motivated to stay active. Using these tips, you can create a routine that fits your lifestyle and will keep you on track for long-term success.

3. Warm-up Exercise and stretches

Warm-up exercises and stretches are physical activities that help to prepare the body for exercise or other physical activities. They help to get the blood flowing, increase heart rate, improve flexibility and range of motion, reduce risk of injury, boost mental focus and alertness, as well as warm up muscles before a workout session.

The importance of warm-up exercises and stretches cannot be overstated. Without them, it is much more likely that you will injure yourself during your workout due to cold muscles which are less elastic than warmed-up muscles. Warming up also helps to gradually increase your heart rate so that you don't experience any sudden shock when starting your actual workout routine. It also helps mentally by getting you in the right frame of mind to exercise.

The best way to warm up is by doing dynamic stretches, which involve moving the muscles that you will be using during your workout. This could include leg swings, arm circles, and torso twists. You should also do some light cardio such as walking or jogging for 5-10 minutes before starting your routine as this will help get your heart rate up and prepare the body for more intense activity.

It's important to remember that a good warm-up should not take longer than 10 minutes so make sure you don't spend too much time on it otherwise you won't have enough energy left for your actual workout session.

Overall, warm-up exercises and stretches are an essential part of any workout routine. They help to reduce the risk of injury and prepare your body for exercise both physically and mentally. Make sure you always spend at least 5-10 minutes warming up before starting your workout.

I. Different types of Stretching Techniques

Stretching is an important component of any exercise or workout routine, as it helps to improve flexibility and range of motion while reducing the risk of injury. There are a variety of different types of stretching techniques that can be used to target specific muscle groups and increase overall mobility.

1. Static Stretching: Static stretching involves holding a stretch for an extended period (typically 15-30 seconds) without moving. This type of stretching is most effective when done after a warm-up, as it increases blood flow to the muscles being stretched and reduces tension in them. Static stretches should not be done before exercise, however, as they may reduce performance due to decreased power output from the muscles being stretched. Examples include toe touches, calf stretches, and shoulder rolls.

2. Dynamic Stretching: Dynamic stretching involves active movements that stretch the muscles without holding them in a static position for an extended period. This type of stretching is best done before exercise, as it warms up the body and increases blood flow to the muscles being stretched. Examples include arm circles, leg swings, and lunges.

3. Ballistic Stretching: Ballistic stretching uses short but intense bouncing motions to stretch a muscle group beyond its normal range of motion. This type of stretching should only be used by experienced exercisers who

understand how their bodies respond to this type of movement; otherwise, it can increase the risk of injury due to overstretching or tearing a muscle group. Examples include bouncing toe touches and calf raises.

4. PNF Stretching: Proprioceptive Neuromuscular Facilitation (PNF) stretching is a type of stretching that combines passive stretching with active contraction of the muscle group being stretched. This type of stretching can help to increase the range of motion more quickly than other types, as it uses both neural pathways and muscular contractions to achieve greater flexibility. PNF stretches typically involve holding a stretch for 8-10 seconds while actively contracting the muscle group being stretched, followed by another 8-10 second hold in which the muscles are relaxed. Examples include assisted hamstring stretches and assisted hip flexor stretches.

5. Yoga: Yoga is an ancient practice that involves postures or poses designed to increase flexibility, strength, and balance. It is a combination of physical postures, breathing

techniques, relaxation, and meditation that can help to improve overall health and well-being. Yoga poses typically involve stretching the muscles in all directions while focusing on proper alignment and breath control. Examples include downward-facing dog, triangle pose, and cobra pose.

II. Basic Stretching Routines For Beginners

Stretching is an important component of any exercise routine, as it helps to improve flexibility, reduce the risk of injury and promote better posture. For beginners who are just starting with a new exercise program, Here are some basic stretching routines that can help them get started safely and effectively.

1. Full-Body Stretch: This stretch involves standing up straight with your feet shoulder-width apart and your arms extended outward in front of you. Gently reach as far forward as possible while keeping your back flat and your head up, then slowly return to the original position. Do this for 10 slow repetitions for a full-body stretch.

2. Hamstring Stretch: To target the hamstrings specifically, stand up straight with your feet shoulder-width apart and one foot slightly ahead of the other. Bend at the waist, keeping your back flat, and reach down to touch your toes (or as far as you can comfortably go). Hold this position for 30 seconds before slowly returning to standing. Do this stretch on both legs.

3. Quadriceps Stretch: To target the quadriceps muscles, stand up straight and hold onto a wall or chair if needed for balance. Lift one leg behind you, grab it just above the ankle with one hand, and pull it towards your buttocks until you feel a gentle stretch in the front of that thigh muscle. Hold this position for 30 seconds before repeating it on the other leg.

4. Chest Stretch: To target the chest muscles, stand up straight and clasp your hands behind you. Raise your arms and gently pull them back towards your body until you feel a gentle stretch in the front of your chest. Hold this position for 30 seconds before releasing softly.

5. Shoulder Stretch: To target the shoulder muscles, stand with one arm crossed over to the opposite side of your body so that it is touching just above or below your armpit. With the other hand, grab onto that elbow and gently pull it away from you while keeping both feet on the ground until you feel a gentle stretch in that shoulder muscle group. Hold this stance for 30 seconds before switching arms and continuing on the other side.

By including these basic stretching routines in your exercise program, you can ensure that your body is adequately prepared for the physical activity ahead and reduce the risk of injury.

4. Cardio Exercise For Beginners

Cardio exercise for beginners is a great way to get into shape and stay healthy. It can help you lose weight, build muscle, increase your energy level, reduce stress levels, and improve your overall health. Cardio exercises are typically any activity that increases your heart rate and breathing rate for an extended period. Common cardio exercises include running, walking, biking, swimming, or using an elliptical machine.

Before starting any type of exercise program it's important to consult with your doctor first. This will ensure that you don't have any underlying medical conditions which could be affected by the intensity of the workout or the duration of it. Once cleared by your doctor, begin slowly with light-intensity workouts such as brisk walking or jogging, then gradually increase the intensity as your body becomes accustomed to it.

When you begin working out, start by warming up with light stretching and deep breathing exercises for a few minutes. This will help loosen tight muscles and reduce the risk of injury during your workout. After warming up, make sure to drink plenty of water before beginning any cardio exercise routine to stay hydrated throughout the session.

The best type of cardio exercise for beginners is low-impact aerobic activity such as walking or biking on flat surfaces rather than running on hills or uneven terrain. Low-impact activities are less strenuous on joints and tendons which makes them easier for those just starting with an exercise program. In addition, many people find these types of activities to be more enjoyable and less intimidating than higher-intensity workouts.

When starting a cardio exercise program, aim for at least 30 minutes of activity a day, five days a week. If you're new to exercising you may want to start with 10-15 minute sessions three times a week and gradually increase the time as your fitness level improves. It's important to listen to your body when performing any type of exercise and take breaks if needed to avoid overexertion.

Cardio exercise for beginners is a great way to get into shape and stay healthy. With consistency, dedication, and the right type of workout program, you can make significant progress in improving your overall health and fitness level. So start slowly, listen to your body, drink plenty of water and enjoy the process!

I.   Running for fitness

Running for fitness is a great way to get in shape, lose weight, and improve overall health. It's an easy form of exercise that anyone can do regardless of their fitness level or age. Running has many benefits including improving cardiovascular health, strengthening the muscles and bones, increasing endurance, burning calories and fat, boosting mental well-being, as well as promoting healthy body composition. For beginners who are just starting with running for fitness, it's important to start slowly and gradually increase the intensity over time. Start by walking at a brisk pace for 10-15 minutes every day then add jogging intervals into your routine when you feel comfortable doing so. Make sure to warm up before each session with light stretching or walking then cool down afterward with more light stretching. In addition to running, it's important to strength train and do other forms of physical activity to maximize the benefits of your fitness routine.

Strength training can help build muscle, increase bone density and improve overall balance, coordination and posture. Other activities such as swimming, biking, or playing sports can also be beneficial for cardiovascular health, flexibility, and agility. Finally, make sure you stay hydrated before during, and after each workout session by drinking plenty of water throughout the day. Eating a healthy diet that is rich in fruits, vegetables, and lean proteins will also provide your body with the essential nutrients needed for optimal performance while exercising. With consistency over time, one should begin to see results from their efforts such as increased energy, improved mood, and better overall health.

II.   Swimming and Water Aerobics

Swimming and water aerobics are great forms of exercise for beginners. Swimming is a low-impact form of exercise that can be beneficial to the body by providing cardiovascular conditioning, strengthening muscles, improving endurance and flexibility, and aiding in weight loss.

Water aerobics is also an effective form of exercise as it uses the resistance provided by the water to strengthen muscles while providing aerobic benefits as well. When first beginning swimming or water aerobics, it is important to start slowly and gradually build up the intensity over time. Beginners should focus on technique rather than speed or distance when starting; proper technique will help reduce injury risk and make swimming more enjoyable. It may be helpful for those just starting to take lessons from an experienced swimmer to learn proper technique. When engaging in water aerobics, beginners should start with basic exercises such as walking or jogging in place and slowly increase intensity as they become more comfortable. Other exercises can include squats, lunges, and arm circles. Adding resistance like dumbbells or ankle weights can also be beneficial for increasing the difficulty of the workout.

The key is to find movements that are challenging yet doable to maximize the benefits of working out while avoiding injury. Swimming and water aerobics provide a great way for beginners to get started on their fitness journey without putting too much strain on their bodies. With proper technique and gradually increased intensity, these forms of exercise can help build strength, increase endurance, and aid in weight loss.

III. Cycling as a Low-impact Exercise

Cycling as a low-impact exercise is an excellent way for beginners to get into shape. Unlike many other forms of exercise, cycling does not require intense physical exertion or high impact on the joints and muscles. As such, it can be easier on the body than running or weight training and can provide a great workout without putting too much strain on the body. One of the main advantages of cycling as a low-impact exercise is that it allows you to work out your entire body while keeping your heart rate up. Cycling requires both lower and upper body movement which helps to strengthen all major muscle groups in your legs, core, arms, back, and chest. It also increases cardiovascular endurance by getting your heart rate up while still providing enough resistance to build strength.

Cycling is also a great way for beginners to get used to the idea of regular exercise without too much strain on their bodies. Many people find that they can gradually increase their intensity and duration as they become more comfortable with the activity, allowing them to work out at an appropriate level for their fitness goals. Additionally, cycling can be done indoors or outdoors so you can adjust your workout based on weather conditions or personal preference. Finally, cycling as a low-impact exercise is relatively inexpensive compared to many other forms of exercise equipment such as treadmills and elliptical machines. This makes it an ideal option for those who may not have access to gym facilities or expensive equipment but still want to get in shape.

Overall, cycling as a low-impact exercise is an excellent way for beginners to get into shape and build strength without putting too much strain on their bodies. It provides a great workout while still allowing you to gradually increase your intensity and duration over time. Additionally, it can be done indoors or outdoors and is relatively inexpensive compared to other forms of exercise equipment.

5. Strength Training Exercise For Beginners

Strength training exercises for beginners are a great way to improve overall health and fitness. Strength training helps build muscle, increase strength, reduce body fat, and boost metabolism. It can also help prevent injury, reduce stress levels and improve posture.

When starting with strength training as a beginner there are some important tips to keep in mind:

- Start slowly - don't try to do too much too soon or you may risk injury
- Choose exercises that use multiple muscle groups at once – this will give you the most bang for your buck
- Focus on compound movements – these involve multiple joints which will help develop coordination and balance as well as building strength
- Make sure you have proper form when doing your exercises – this will ensure you are using the correct muscles and not putting too much strain on any one area

- Use a variety of different exercises to work all parts of the body
- Incorporate rest days into your workout plan so that your body can recover properly
- Begin with lighter weights and work your way up as you gain strength.

Some great strength training exercises for beginners include squats, lunges, push-ups, pull-ups, bicep curls, and triceps dips. These exercises target multiple muscle groups at once which makes them ideal for beginner workouts. Additionally, they are compound movements that help develop coordination and balance while building strength. With proper form, these exercises can be done safely with minimal risk of injury or strain.

Strength training is an important part of any fitness plan and can help to improve overall health, reduce stress levels, increase strength and build muscle. For beginners, it's important to start slowly and use proper form when doing exercises. Incorporating a variety of compound movements that target multiple muscle groups will give you the most bang for your buck while helping to prevent injury. With these tips in mind, anyone can begin their journey towards improved fitness with strength training exercises for beginners.

I.   Bodyweight Exercise to Build Muscle

Bodyweight exercises are an effective and convenient way to build muscle, as they require no additional equipment or gym membership. This type of exercise is ideal for beginners who don't have access to a gym yet want to get in shape and increase their strength.

Using only your body weight for resistance provides enough challenge for the average person looking to build muscle without having to buy any complicated machines or weights. The basic premise of these exercises involves using gravity as a source of resistance by pushing or pulling against it with your body weight. To maximize results and make each exercise more challenging, it's important to focus on proper form and technique. Start by performing the exercises slowly and in a controlled manner, focusing on using a good form rather than speed or how many reps you can do at once.

It is also beneficial to increase the difficulty of your bodyweight exercises over time as your muscles grow stronger and become more accustomed to the movements. This can be done by adding weight (e.g., wearing a weighted vest) or increasing the number of reps per set. Additionally, varying the types of exercises used will help keep things interesting while still providing an effective workout routine for muscle-building purposes.

Here are a few bodyweight exercises that can help you get started:

1. Push-Ups: Push-ups are one of the most fundamental bodyweight exercises out there and they work the chest, shoulders, triceps, and core muscles all at once. To do a push-up properly make sure to keep your arms slightly wider than shoulder-width apart with your palms flat on the ground or floor. Keep your back straight as you lower yourself towards the ground until your chest is just above it before pushing yourself back up again for one rep.

2. Squats: Squats target both legs but focus more on the glutes and quads. To do a squat correctly, stand with your feet slightly wider than shoulder-width apart. Push your hips back and bend at the knees while keeping

your chest up until your thighs are parallel to the ground before pushing yourself back up again for one rep.

3. Lunges: Lunges target both legs but focus more on the glutes and hamstrings than squats do. To do a lunge properly, start by standing with feet slightly wider than shoulder-width apart then take a big step forward with one foot as you lower down towards the ground ensuring that both of your knees form 90-degree angles when done correctly you should be able to tap the floor lightly with the knee of your front leg before pushing yourself back up again for one rep.

4. Pull-Ups: Pull-ups are excellent exercises for building upper body strength and can be done with or without equipment. To do a pull-up properly, grab onto the bar with your hands slightly wider than shoulder width apart before pulling yourself up until your chin is above the bar then lower back down again for one rep.

5. Plank: Planks are an amazing core exercise that works all of the muscles in the midsection from front to back at once. To do

a plank correctly start by laying on your stomach then prop yourself up on your elbows keeping them directly beneath your shoulders while making sure to keep your spine straight and feet together as you hold this position for 30 seconds before repeating it for multiple sets.

These are just a few bodyweight exercises that can help you build muscle and strength while also increasing your cardiovascular endurance. With consistency and proper form, these exercises will help you achieve the results you desire in no time!

II. Using Free Weights To Strengthen Muscles

Using free weights to strengthen muscles is an effective way for beginners to exercise and build muscle. Free weights are relatively inexpensive and can be used at home or in the gym, making them a great option for those just starting on their fitness journey.

When using free weights, it's important to start with lighter weights (2-5 lbs) and focus on proper form before increasing the amount of weight you lift.

Using proper form will help ensure that you are targeting the right muscles while also avoiding injury. You should focus on slow, controlled movements when lifting any type of weight so that your body has time to adjust and become stronger as you progress.

Free weights typically come in two forms – barbells and dumbbells. Barbells and dumbbells are two of the most common pieces of equipment used in exercise and working out for beginners. Barbells are large metal bars with weight plates attached to each end. They come in a variety of sizes, ranging from light weights for beginners up to heavy weights for experienced lifters.

Dumbbells, on the other hand, consist of two separate metal handles connected by a short bar that allows users to hold them comfortably while lifting. Both barbells and dumbbells can be used for a wide range of exercises such as squats, deadlifts, presses, and rows. Barbell exercises involve using both arms or legs simultaneously which is great for developing overall strength and muscle size since it requires more effort from the body. Barbells also allow for a greater range of motion, enabling users to target specific muscle groups more effectively. They are great for compound exercises such as squats, deadlifts, and overhead presses which involve multiple joints and muscles at once. Dumbbell exercises on the other hand require only one arm or leg to be used at a time. This makes them perfect for training smaller muscle groups like biceps or triceps as well as focusing on balance and stability during single-arm movements like lateral raises or lunges. Dumbbells can also be used in combination with barbell exercises by adding extra resistance to heavier lifts such as bench presses or squats.

When using free weights it's important to start slow and focus on form before increasing the amount of weight lifted. Doing so will help ensure that your muscles become stronger in a safe way while also avoiding injury. As your strength increases over time, gradually increase the amount of weight you lift until eventually reach your desired level of fitness.

Some exercises that are great for beginners include bicep curls, triceps extensions, chest presses, and shoulder presses. These exercises can be done with either barbells or dumbbells and will help to strengthen the muscles in your arms, chest, and shoulders. Additionally, squats, deadlifts, and lunges can also be used to target the muscles in your legs. Using free weights is an effective way for beginners to exercise and build muscle strength. It's important to start slow by focusing on the form before increasing the amount of weight lifted over time as you become stronger. Doing so will help ensure that you get the maximum benefit from each exercise while avoiding injury at the same time!

II. Resistance Band Training Basics

Resistance band training is a great way to get into shape and strengthen your muscles. It's easy to use, cost-effective and can be done just about anywhere. Plus, it offers an effective workout with minimal equipment needed.
The basic premise of resistance band training is the same as any other type of strength training: The bands provide resistance against which you must work to build muscle strength and tone. Resistance bands come in various levels of tension so that you can gradually increase the intensity as you progress through your workouts.
When using a resistance band for exercise, begin by choosing one that fits snugly around both hands or

feet (depending on what exercise you are doing). Make sure there's enough tension in the band to provide resistance, but not so much that it's uncomfortable.

Once you have your band in place, start by performing basic exercises like bicep curls and triceps extensions. These are simple movements that can be done with just about any type of exercise equipment or even bodyweight exercises. Start with slow, controlled motions and gradually increase the speed as you become more comfortable with the movement. You should also focus on keeping your form correct throughout each rep for maximum benefit from the exercise.

As you progress through your workout routine, try incorporating other types of exercises using a resistance band such as squats, deadlifts, rows, and overhead presses. As always keep good form when doing these exercises and focus on the muscles being targeted.

One of the great things about resistance band training is that it can be done anywhere, anytime. This makes it perfect for those who don't have access to a gym or other fitness equipment and even those with limited space in their home. Plus, you can add more tension as your strength increases so that you are always pushing yourself to new levels.

6. Cool Down Routines and Recovery Strategies

Cool-down routines and recovery strategies refer to the activities that athletes do after training or competition to reduce muscle fatigue, prevent injury, and promote relaxation. Cooling down is an important part of any exercise program because it helps your muscles recover from intense physical activity.

A proper cool-down routine should begin with light aerobic exercises like walking or jogging for 5-10 minutes at a slower pace than the workout. This can help bring your heart rate back to normal levels while also allowing lactic acid (a byproduct of exercise) to be cleared from your muscles.

Next, stretching can help improve flexibility and range of motion in your joints as well as decrease soreness and tightness in the muscles you just worked out. Static stretches are best for cooling down since they involve holding a position for an extended period. Finally, breathing exercises can help relax the body and reduce stress levels. Recovery strategies are also important for athletes to incorporate into their regular training programs to prevent injury and promote optimal performance. After a workout or competition, it is important to take some time to rest and recover before the next session. This could include getting adequate sleep (7-9 hours per night), eating nutritious meals throughout the day, drinking plenty of water, using foam rollers or other self-massage tools on sore muscles, taking ice baths/cold showers after workouts that were particularly intense, and doing light active recovery such as walking or swimming at low-intensity levels. All these strategies can help reduce fatigue, improve performance, and prevent injuries.

Overall, cool-down routines and recovery strategies are essential components of any athlete's training program. They can help reduce muscle fatigue and soreness while also preventing injury and promoting relaxation. Taking the time to properly cool down after exercise and incorporating various recovery strategies into your routine is key for optimal performance in any sport.

I.   Post-Workout Stretching Techniques

Post-workout stretching techniques are an important part of any exercise routine for beginners. Not only does stretching help to reduce soreness and improve flexibility, but it can also be beneficial in helping to prevent injury.

For most exercises, the best post-workout stretch is a dynamic one. This means that instead of holding each stretch for a set amount of time, you move through them quickly as your muscles warm up after exercising. For example, if you just finished running or biking, you might do some walking stretches like lunges or high knees with arm swings before getting into more static stretches (holding a position) like touching your toes or side splits.

When doing static stretches after working out, hold each pose for at least 30 seconds, and try to focus on deep breathing as you stretch. This helps relax the body and increases flexibility.

When stretching after a strength-training session, it's important to target both the muscles used in your workout and opposing muscles that may be tight from being underused. For example, if you just finished doing squats or lunges, be sure to also do stretches for your hip flexors (the front of your hips). It's also essential to make sure you are using the proper form when stretching. If something feels uncomfortable or painful, stop immediately and modify the position until it is more comfortable. Be sure not to push yourself too hard; post-workout stretching should feel good rather than painful. Finally, it's important to listen to your body and not overdo it with stretching after a workout. Too much stretching can be detrimental if done improperly or too often. It is best to focus on dynamic stretches that warm up the muscles before doing more static stretches, and try not to stretch for longer than 30 seconds per muscle group.

II. Tips on Developing an Effective Cool Down Routine

Developing an effective cool-down regimen is a vital aspect of any beginner's workout. A cool-down helps your body transition from exercise to rest and reduces the risk of injury or soreness after a workout. Here are some tips on developing an effective cool-down routine:

1. Start with light stretching: Light stretching is a great way to start your cool down because it helps reduce tension in the muscles you used during your workout and can help improve flexibility over time. Start by taking deep breaths while lightly stretching each muscle group in the order that they were worked out - this will help relax them more quickly. Make sure not to stretch too far as this could cause further damage, instead just focus on holding each stretch for 10-30 seconds.

2. Incorporate foam rolling: Foam rolling is an effective way to help reduce muscle soreness and improve circulation in the muscles you worked out during your session. Start by slowly moving a foam roller over each muscle group, focusing on areas that feel particularly tight or sore. You can use a tennis ball instead if you don't have access to a foam roller as this will also help break down knots and tension in the muscles.

3. Use heat packs: Heat packs are great for helping warm up the muscles after a workout, which can help reduce post-workout stiffness and soreness. Place them on any areas of your

body that feel particularly tight or uncomfortable and let them sit for 10-15 minutes.

4. Finish with breathing exercises: Breathing exercises are a great way to help your body relax and transition from exercise to rest. Start by focusing on your breath - take slow, deep breaths in through the nose and out through the mouth for 5-10 minutes. This will help reduce stress levels, improve circulation, and restore balance in the body after an intense workout session.

5. Listen to your body: Lastly, it's important to always listen to your body and adjust your cool-down routine accordingly. If any areas feel particularly sore or tight after a workout, take the time to stretch them out further or use a foam roller for extra relief. This will help reduce tension in those areas and ultimately improve your performance over time.

By following these tips, you can create an effective cool-down routine that will help you recover more quickly from workouts and reduce any post-workout soreness or stiffness. Implementing a cool down into your workout routine is essential for beginners as it helps prevent injury while also aiding in recovery time so that you can get back to working out sooner.

II.   Tips on Recovering After Intense Workouts

Recovering after intense workouts is an essential part of any exercise and working out routine. It allows your body to rest, repair, and rebuild so that you can perform at a high level during future workouts. Here are some tips on how to properly recover after intensive exercise:

1. Hydrate: Make sure to drink plenty of fluids before, during, and after your workout session as dehydration can lead to fatigue and muscle soreness. Additionally, electrolyte-rich beverages such as coconut water or sports drinks can help replenish lost minerals from sweat.

2. Eat Well: Eating nutrient-dense foods like lean proteins (chicken breast), complex carbs (brown rice), and healthy fats (avocado) after an intense workout can help replenish energy stores and promote muscle recovery.

3. Rest: After a strenuous workout, it's important to give your body time to rest and recover. Take at least one full day off from training each week and aim for 8-9 hours of sleep per night to ensure you are well-rested before your next session.

4. Active Recovery: Low-intensity activities such as walking, swimming, or yoga can help promote recovery without putting too much strain on the body. These activities help increase circulation, reduce inflammation and flush out lactic acid built up in the muscles during intense workouts.

Recovery is a key component of any workout routine, so make sure to take time to properly rest and recover after each session. Following these tips will ensure that you are well-prepared for your next workout and minimize injury risk over time.

7. Nutrition & Healthy Eating Habits

Nutrition and healthy eating habits are essential components of a successful fitness program, especially for those just starting to exercise. Eating nutritious foods provides the body with the energy and nutrients it needs to perform at its best during workouts, as well as helps promote muscle growth and recovery afterward. Establishing good nutrition habits is key to helping beginners reach their fitness goals.

When it comes to nutrition, there are no one-size-fits-all solutions; instead, each individual should strive to create an eating plan that works best for them. However, some general guidelines can be helpful when developing an effective diet plan:

1. Eat plenty of fruits and vegetables - Fruits and veggies provide vitamins, minerals, fiber, and other important nutrients that the body needs to stay healthy and energized. Additionally, they are low in calories, making them perfect for those looking to lose weight.

2. Choose lean proteins - Lean sources of protein such as chicken, fish, eggs, and legumes provide the building blocks for muscle growth and repair. They also help keep you feeling full longer between meals.

3. Limit processed foods - Processed foods can be high in sugar, fat, and sodium – all of which can contribute to weight gain if eaten in excess. Instead, opt for minimally processed whole foods whenever possible.

4. Drink plenty of water - Staying hydrated is important when exercising; it helps your muscles work efficiently while also aiding digestion and keeping toxins flushed from the body. Aim to consume 8-10 glasses of water every day.

5. Get enough sleep - Getting adequate rest is essential for muscle recovery, energy levels, and overall well-being. Aim to get 7-8 hours of quality sleep each night to maximize your fitness results.

In addition to following a healthy diet plan, beginners should also strive to establish good eating habits that will help them maintain their progress long-term. Eating smaller meals more frequently

(3-4 times per day) helps keep blood sugar levels stable and prevents overeating at mealtime; it also keeps energy levels high throughout the day which can be especially beneficial when exercising regularly. Additionally, planning meals ahead of time ensure you have access to nutritious foods when needed and also helps you stick to your diet plan.

Nutrition is an important part of any fitness program, but especially for beginners who are just starting. Eating a balanced diet that includes plenty of fruits and vegetables, lean proteins, complex carbohydrates, and healthy fats will provide the energy and nutrients needed to support workouts while helping promote muscle growth and recovery afterward. Establishing good eating habits such as smaller meals more frequently throughout the day can further help beginners stay on track with their nutrition goals to maximize their results from exercise.

I. The Importance of Eating Right

Eating right is an essential part of any exercise and working out program for beginners. It may seem daunting to try to figure out what you should be eating, but it's important to understand the basics to make sure you are getting all the nutrients your body needs. Proper nutrition helps ensure that your body has enough energy for workouts, aids in recovery after physical activity, and can even help boost performance during exercise.

The first step when it comes to eating right is understanding how much food you need. This will depend on several factors such as age, sex, height, weight, and activity level. Generally speaking, women require around 2200 calories per day while men typically need 2500-3000 calories per day depending on their activity level. Understanding how many calories you need can help you plan your meals and snacks accordingly.

It's also important to make sure that your diet is balanced. That means eating a variety of foods from each of the five food groups: fruits, vegetables, grains, proteins, and dairy products. Eating a wide variety of foods helps ensure that you are getting all the vitamins, minerals and other nutrients your body needs for optimal health and performance during exercise. It's also important to drink plenty of water throughout the day as this will help keep you hydrated so that your muscles have enough energy for workouts and recovery afterward.

In addition to eating healthy, it's also important to pay attention to when you eat. Eating a small snack before and after exercise can help provide the energy you need for workouts. It's also important to eat meals at regular intervals throughout the day to ensure that your body has enough fuel for physical activity.

Finally, it's important to remember that proper nutrition is an ongoing process. As your activity level increases and you become more physically fit, you may need to adjust your diet accordingly to make sure that you are getting all the nutrients your body needs. This may require consulting with a registered dietitian or nutritionist who can help develop an eating plan tailored specifically to your individual needs and goals. Eating right is essential for anyone looking to get into shape through exercise and working out.

II. Tips on Eating Healthy

Eating healthy is a key component of any exercise and working out routine. Healthy eating habits provide the fuel your body needs to sustain activity, as well as provide essential nutrients that are necessary for overall health and well-being. Here are some tips on how to eat healthier when starting an exercise program:

1. Eat more fruits and vegetables: Fruits and vegetables contain important vitamins, minerals, antioxidants, fiber, and other nutrients that help keep your body strong and energized during physical activity. Aim to fill half of your plate with fresh produce at each meal or snack.

2. Choose lean proteins: Protein helps build muscle strength while providing energy for workouts; it also helps you stay fuller and longer so you don't feel hungry and tired during exercise. Choose lean proteins like fish, poultry, beans, and legumes for the most health benefits.

3. Opt for whole grains: Whole grains are an excellent source of complex carbohydrates

which provide energy to fuel your workout and help replenish glycogen stores after a hard workout. Examples include oatmeal, quinoa, brown rice, or barley.

4. Watch portion sizes: It's important to eat enough to meet your body's needs but also be mindful not to overeat as this can lead to weight gain if you don't burn off the extra calories with physical activity. Use smaller plates and bowls at meals so that you get used to eating smaller portions without feeling deprived or hungry.

5. Eat healthy fats: Eating healthy fats can help you feel satisfied and provide essential nutrients for good health. Sources of healthy fats include avocados, nuts, seeds, and fatty fish like salmon or mackerel.

6. Drink plenty of water: Staying hydrated is important before, during, and after exercise as it helps keep your energy levels up and prevents dehydration which will make you feel fatigued during physical activity. Aim to drink 6-8 glasses per day (more if exercising in hot weather).

7. Don't forget snacks: Eating small snacks throughout the day can help keep your energy levels up between meals so that you have enough fuel to power through workouts without feeling tired or sluggish. Good snack options include a piece of fruit, nuts or seeds, yogurt, or a few whole-grain crackers. Eating healthy is an important part of any exercise and working out routine. By following these tips you can ensure that your body has the fuel it needs to get the most out of your workouts and stay energized throughout the day.

III. How to Create a Balanced Diet

Creating a balanced diet for exercise and working out is important to ensure you are getting the right nutrients, vitamins, and minerals to fuel your body. A well-rounded diet should include all major food groups: proteins, carbohydrates, fruits & vegetables, dairy products, and healthy fats.

- Proteins: Proteins play an essential role in muscle growth and repair. Eating lean sources of protein such as chicken, turkey, fish or eggs will help provide your body with the necessary building blocks it needs for muscle development. Additionally adding nuts or seeds can also help boost protein intake.

- Carbohydrates: Carbohydrates provide energy for physical activity so having enough of them is important if you are exercising regularly. Whole grains like oats, quinoa, and brown rice are good sources of complex carbohydrates that will provide sustained energy. Additionally adding some fruits to your diet as well can help boost carbohydrate intake.
- Fruits & Vegetables: Eating a variety of fruits and vegetables is important for overall health and wellness. Fruits like apples, oranges, and bananas provide essential vitamins and minerals while vegetables such as spinach, kale, and broccoli contain fiber which helps keep you full longer. Aim to have at least one serving of fruit or vegetables with each meal or snack throughout the day.
- Dairy Products: Dairy products such as milk, yogurt, or cheese are great sources of calcium which is important for strong bones as well as

muscle contraction during exercise. Low-fat dairy options should be chosen as they are lower in calories and saturated fat.

- Healthy Fats: Healthy fats like avocados, nuts, and seeds provide essential fatty acids that the body needs for proper functioning. Eating healthy fats can also help reduce inflammation which is important for muscle recovery after a workout.

In addition to eating the right types of foods, portion control is also important when creating a balanced diet for exercise and working out. Aim to fill half your plate with fruits & vegetables while splitting the other half between proteins, carbohydrates, and healthy fats. This will ensure you are getting all of the necessary nutrients without overindulging in calories or unhealthy foods. Finally, it's key to stay hydrated throughout the day by drinking lots of water.

By following these simple steps you can create a balanced diet for exercise and working out that will provide your body with the essential nutrients it needs to stay healthy and energized.

8. Conclusion

Congratulations on completing Get Fit Now!: A Beginner's Guide to Exercising and Working Out. You have taken the first step to a healthier and happier you.

By now, you should have a better understanding of how to begin exercising and working out. You have learned about the importance of warming up and cooling down the different types of exercise equipment, the importance of proper nutrition, and the benefits of tracking your progress. Through this book, you have gained the knowledge and confidence to make good choices when it comes to your fitness journey.

The world of exercise and fitness can be intimidating at first, but it can also be incredibly rewarding. It is important to remember to start slow and gradually increase your intensity as you become more comfortable and confident with your routine. Exercise is not only beneficial for your physical well-being but also for your mental and emotional health. The endorphins released during exercise will help to reduce stress, improve your mood, and give you a sense of accomplishment.

It is important to stay motivated and consistent with your fitness goals. Take time to appreciate your progress and celebrate your successes. If you find yourself struggling to stay motivated, consider working with a personal trainer or joining a fitness class. Set realistic goals for yourself and remember to have fun!

I hope that this book has been a helpful resource in your journey to becoming fit and healthy. Best of luck to you on your fitness journey!

9 798373 135931